'The Way of Yoga'

Yogacharyia Jnandev

Publisher
Design Marque

'The Way of Yoga'

Copyright © Yogacharyia Jnandev 2009

All Rights Reserved

No part of this book may be reproduced in any form,
by photocopying or by any electronic or mechanical means,
Including information storage or retrieval systems,
without permission in writing from both the copyright
owner and the publisher of this book

First Published 2010

Second Edition 2016
ISBN 978-0-9927841-6-4

Printed in Great Britain
by
Design Marque

Editors Note

Yogacharyia Jnandev is a well accomplished Yoga teacher. He began his yoga journey through first studying a master's degree in Preksha Meditation and Yoga in the Jain Vishwa Bharati University Rajasthan where he excelled and obtained the 'gold medal' award upon completion, recognition of being the best student in the university. He spent several years after this teaching Yoga in schools in India and working in community projects for disadvantaged and vulnerable people, using tools of Yoga to improve the lives of others. He also spent a great deal of time travelling around India staying in different Ashrams and learning different styles of Yoga and studying under various Swamiji's and Sadhus. Surender has spent time not only learning but also practicing the techniques he has learnt, he has spend time in solitude in regions of the Himalayas and other parts of India to try to understand and realise the deeper meanings of Yoga.

He has recently settled in West Wales, UK and is in the process of establishing a Yoga Ashram, to benefit sincere Yoga Practitioners to come, learn and practice Yoga in a yogic environment.

Yogacharini Deepika
Yoga Satsanga Ashram, Wales
December 2009

Dedication

All of my ideas, thoughts and understandings about yoga and life are enriched by the teachings of Amma Meenakshi Devi, Dr Ananda and Devasana of Ananda Ashram, Puducherry, India. This book is basically based on all the aspects of yoga I have learned from various yoga and spiritual masters, literatures and institution, I am sincerely grateful to all of them to guide me on yoga path. I am grateful to God for keeping me surrounded with loving and caring family and friends.

I am grateful to all my yoga students who keep me uplifted and motivated for teaching and reconstructing my ideas and thoughts of yogic life in western life style. I am thankful to Sarah Ray for bringing this book together with her designing skills. I am also thankful to Ange Smith and my mother in law Carol Forde for helping with proof reading. Love and thanks for all their sincere efforts!

Finally it all goes to my better-half (ardhangini in Hindi) who is guiding me in every moment of my life since we are together after our marriage. She has done the actual work of bringing my ideas together, editing and discussing and I would like her to re-write it at some point for all of us.

Lots of love for our little one Siddha full of energy and blessing us by being with me in our daily classes and bringing more light and joy into our lives!

Yogacharyia Jnandev
Yoga Satsanga Ashram, Wales
December 2009

Introduction

This book is written for the Yoga sadhaka (aspirant), who is seeking to know something more of Yoga, what its roots are, where posture work fits in to the greater picture of the complete science of Yoga, as apposed to being the only purpose of Yoga. Many of the deeper philosophies and basics of yogic philosophy are addressed in this short book. It is written in a way that is easy to understand for those without any previous study of Yoga, but contains a great deal on higher concepts for the more experienced yoga practitioner to contemplate.

The foundations of the yogi or yogini's spiritual life, moral and ethical considerations are addressed here, in addition to this other forms of yoga are looked at briefly for the reader to gain some insight into the great world of yoga and how the worlds people have developed different strains of perhaps India's greatest gift, the origins of yoga. Hinduism in ancient times was very intertwined with Yogic life, as its path requires a disciplined pure lifestyle in its most refined form. When we study yoga at its roots, it is important to have some insights into ancient Hindu lifestyle which this book will include.

One of the aims of this work is to give those who already practice Yoga to develop their awareness into the higher aspects of Yoga and refine their physical practice. Yoga is essentially a tool for self development and furthermore a path to unite with the 'one' that makes up this entire universe - Yoga literally means 'union'.

I hope this book will allow you to reflect and think about your life, spiritual journey and Yoga as it has for us.

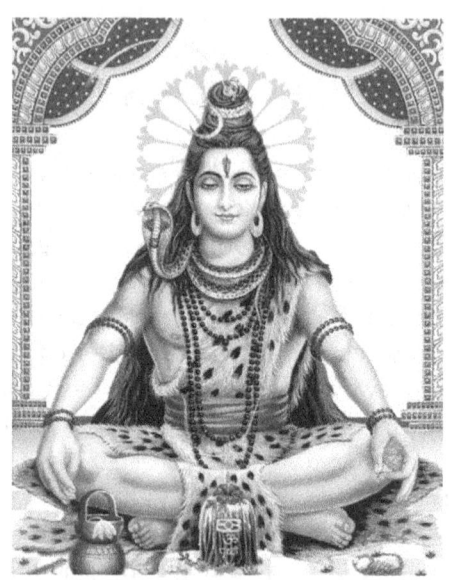

Contents

What is Yoga?	7
Yamas or Restraints	16
Niyamas or Duties to be adhered for evolution	20
Hatha-Yoga Concepts and benefits of Asanas	25
Pranayama or the Science of Vital Energy	28
Prana, thoughts and emotions	34
Prana philosophical Aspects	35
How to meditate	40
Yoga uniting the self and Supreme-self	45
Glossary	47

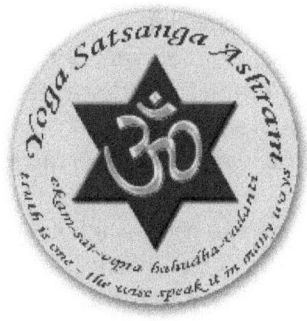

What is Yoga?

"Yoga is the science of the sciences. Yoga is an art, a philosophy, a religion, a fad and a fanaticism." The Meaning or definition of yoga depends on the individual person, according to their level of consciousness and evolution. Yoga can be simply described as the process to control the perception and the conceptions, which develop the conscious, rational thinking and viveka (discernment).

Yoga is one of most precious jewels of the Ancient Hindu ways of attaining liberation. Even then yoga is not concerned with religion. Yoga can help us to live with greater harmony. Today you can find people practicing yoga everywhere. Hatha-Yoga (Asanas and Pranayama) has become the synonym of yoga. So to enhance the meaning of your life, religion, faith and practices, yoga is the tool, which is free from religion, cast or creed, available for one and all.

The term 'Yoga', which is multivalent and derived from the root 'yuj', generally means 'union', 'to join', 'to yoke together', or 'to unite as one'. The word yoga comes from the most ancient language known to man Sanskrita. In India, Sanskrit is considered to be the language of God, and is formed in a mathematical way.

Yoga in India is also considered as one of the six Ancient Indian Philosophies. Primarily we should keep in mind that yoga is the 'way of union'.

The Bhagavat-Geeta uses it (i.i.48) to mean sole desire for supreme divinity (paramesvarikaparata- sridharasvamin).

In i.i. 50 of the same treatise, yoga denotes skill in work (karmasu kausalam). In IV. 1,2,3, Yoga means Karma yoga (desire less action) and Jnanayoga (acquisition of wisdom; truth and reality).

In VI. 16, 17, the term yoga means Samadhi in which the mind is united with the Atman.

In VI. 23, yoga means a state of mind, which having realized the Supreme Being, is not disturbed even by great suffering.

In i.i. 48 and vi. 33, 36, yoga means samatva or equanimity, i.e., indifference to pleasure and pain.

Yoga can be accepted as a way of life, a way of integrating your whole awareness with the true nature of the Self. Physical, mental, emotional and spiritual aspects of your life should work in integrated harmony with each other.

In arithmetic, 'yoga' means addition. In astronomy it means conjunction, lucky conjunction and also conjunctions that may warn of danger, etc.

In the Upanishads, yoga generally means union; union of Jivatman (soul) with Parmatman (supreme soul).

Patanjali in his Yoga Sutra (i.2) defines yoga as **"yogah-chittavratti-nirodhah"**, this means 'to control of the whirlpools of the mind is yoga'. By yoga, Patanjali means the effort to attain union, or oneness of Self with the Supreme Self.

What is union? In the normal sense of yoga this union means harmony of body, mind, emotions and spirit. It is living in the present, moving and accepting all situations as they are with a positive attitude.

The Devata-Smati says

"visayebhyo nivartyabhi-preterthe manasovasthapanam yogah".
Yoga means fixing the mind on the desired object.

According to Daksha-Smriti, yoga is as follows:
 **"vrittihinam manah krtva ksetrajnahparmatmani
 ekikrtya vimucyate yoganam mukhya ucyate."**

One who is aware of the soul, having turned the mind, which is rendered devoid of function, solely to the Supreme Soul, is liberated; this is called principal yoga.

The Vishnupurana defines yoga:
> "atman-prayatna-sapeksa visista ya manogatih,
> tasya brahamani samyoga yoga ityabhidhiyate."

The connection of that special course of mind, which depends upon ones own effort, with Brahma (The Creator) is called yoga.

Yoga- Scope and Classification

Yoga is broadly divided as Raja yoga and Hatha yoga. The former is concerned mainly with the mind and deals with various processes for controlling and calming it. Hatha yoga is concerned mainly with the body and deals with various means of keeping it fit. Several others are Mantra yoga, Laya yoga, Tantra yoga, Transcendental Meditation, Preksha Meditation, Vipsyana, etc.

1. Raja-Yoga: - Raja yoga of Patanjali, contains much of the teachings of the other systems. It aims for the self-realisation of the true nature of Purusha as absolutely distinct from Prakriti.

2. Hatha-Yoga: - It is regarded as preparatory for the practice of Raja yoga. Hatha Yoga is also a system of preventive and therapeutic asanas, kriyas, mudras and pranayamas. The term Hatha is a combination of Ha (prana) and Tha (apana). Lord Shiva in the Shiva Samhita states of 84 million asanas.

3. Mantra-Yoga: - It is the yoga of the act of repetition. This does not teach the mechanical recital of mantras. These must be preceded by earnest solitude to attain the goal and clear knowledge about the meaning of mantras. This is closely connected with the Bhakti-Yoga. The Sandilya Upanishad may be taken as a work on Mantra-Yoga. The Sivasamhita deals with the importance of mantra in practice of Yoga.

4. Laya-Yoga: - It is the yoga of absorption (laya) of mind. The Samadhi has the final aim of the realization of the identity of the finite with the supreme spirit.

5. Tantra Yoga: - Tantra yoga combines elements of both the Raja-Yoga and Hatha-Yoga with a stronger leaning towards the latter. It advocates yoga not only of meditation, but also of action. This exercise balances physical, mental and pranic/ psychic energies.

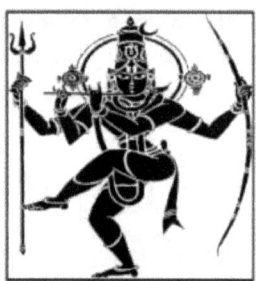

In Tantra there is no difference between Sakti (energy) and Tattva (element) so that Sakti overcomes all obstacles and brings about the unions of the yogi (yoga practitioner) with Supreme Siva. The Tantric Sadhana succeeds in weaving the microcosm and the macrocosm into a single fabric.

6. Karma Yoga: - Yoga of desireless karma (niskam - karman); Union through the action without desire. According to Swami Vivekananda, "He who goes through the streets of a big city with all the traffic and his mind is as calm as if he was in a cave, where not a sound was able to reach him; he is intensely working all the time".

7. Jnana Yoga: - Yoga of right knowledge; union through knowledge. It has three successive stages;
1. Viveka- discrimination between the real and non-real.
2. Vairagya- indifference towards worldly knowledge, joy and sorrow.
3. Mukti- liberation or union with Atman.

The yogin of the Advait Vedanta possess through successive stages in training;
- Sravana-listening,
- Manana- reflection on and analysis of what has been learnt
- Nidhidhyasana- constant and profound meditation.

8. Bhakti Yoga: - In Bhakti-yoga, one devotes himself to his chosen deity to whose honour and glory every action of him is directed. According to Swami

Vivekanada- "He has not to suppress any single one of his emotions; he only strives to intensify them and direct them to God". Bhakti yoga has two stages, one preparatory and other devotional.

9. Kundalini Yoga:- This includes deep study of the energy centres in the body known as the chakras. Each chakra has its own characters, shapes, color, odour, and bija (seed) sounds. The purpose of kundalini yoga is to awaken the serpent power to attain the Samadhi or moksha (freedom or liberation). This includes many kriyas, asanas, mudras, pranayamas and the chanting of bija mantras.

10. Pranayama Yoga: - Only a few pranayamas are included in traditional Hatha yoga. This school of yoga deals with controlling the prana, or the life vital force. They believe prana as the source of life. There aim is also to activate the inactive energy sleeping in the form of the Kundalini.
However, the Gitananda Rishiculture Yoga teaches over 100 pranayamas which should be practiced only after cleansing and a group of breath correcting asanas called the Hathenas.

World Wide Yoga – Way of Life

At this time yoga has become a world-wide philosophy or way of life. But now yoga has become the synonym of some asanas and pranayamas. Some are using yoga as therapy while others are using yoga as the tool of beautification or weight loss, making bodies slim and fit.

Traditionally Yoga is one of the Indian shat-darshanas, or six ways of viewing life. Each of them is accepted as one of the forms of Hinduism. In ancient times Hinduism was not considered a religion, but a way of life. In yoga life there is no conflict of religion, philosophy or science.

Many of the modern yoga schools and Yoga teachers would be wise to re-think Yoga - its actual meanings and importance. Accepting yoga merely as the materialistic tool for physical control is only one drop in the ocean, yet we cannot understand the ocean from one drop. Yoga is the science of life and spirit; yoga is a spiritual way of life aimed to attain self-realization, and conscious evolution of the self. Yoga is discovering the relation of the soul with the Supreme Soul.

Yoga also describes and explains that we each are Self, or the soul and have the capacity to unite with the supreme self. Thus we all possess the capacity to become one with God.
This is one of the reasons of the universal acceptance of yoga as developing the oneness between all living beings on this earth without differentiating them with cast, creed, and colour.

Yoga is highly ethical as the foundation of yoga life begins with the perfection of five yamas, or restraints.
These are breifly:

- Ahimsa, non-violence;
- Satya, adherence to the truth;
- Asteya, non-stealing;
- Brahmacharya, control of sensuality;
- Aparigraha, non-greed.

Yoga is also highly intellectual as it gives full play to the inquiring mind. It describes all the obstacles and distractions and gives complete detail to overcome them through the yoga sutras of Patanjali. Niyamas or observances are given to deal with the body and mind.
These are:
- Saucha, cleanliness;
- Santosha, mental serenity;
- Tapas, discipline and austerities;
- Swadhyaya, self study;
- Isvar-pranidhana, surrender to the supreme self.

Yoga is also scientific as many of its practices, kriyas and prakriyas can be evaluated through scientific experimentation - many medical studies have been done in the field of Yoga.

Yoga as Four-fold Awareness

Our Ancient Rishis, Sadhus or Saints taught that oneness already exists, but that we are unaware of this state of union. So we see duality and multiplicity everywhere. Most of our awareness is diverted to search out the differences between one and another in place of seeing unity. Our yoga approach is to attain that Advaitaik, or state of non-duality.

Yoga is conscious evolution. Our evolution rests in our own hands and it must be conscious, through sensitive awareness. Thus the yamas and niyamas must be learned consciously. Initially you may start with the gross awareness of the body and later on turn to the awareness of the mind and emotions. It may become too strenuous for you to know your own true self-image in beginning.

Yoga teaches a fourfold awareness. The first stage is awareness of the body and how it works, how to care for it, how to love it, how to worship it. That is why in Yoga we often hear, 'our body is our temple' as it is our offering to God. We all want to be healthy and fit – why then are we not? We are living with unawareness in regard to our health, or cannot make the necessary efforts required! Only health begets health. Try to develop the consciousness about right healthy diet, right exercise, right breathing, right rest and relaxation. This includes the complete awareness of all your physical activities going on continuously. This is a type of lifestyle that requires constant training of the mind, to remind us to look after our body every moment, making the right choices for our good health and happiness.

The second stage is awareness of the effect of the emotions upon the body. Most of us are indulged in negative and destructive emotions. Try to be aware of them and their destructive effects on your body and spiralling deterioration of your mental equanimity.

Hate, anger, lust, greed, aversion, envy, irritation, etc are causes of all the psychosomatic diseases, which result in serious illness. Destructive emotions have a powerful detrimental effect upon the body.

Serenity, love, compassion, empathy, understanding, etc have a powerful positive effect on our body; Positive emotions have a beneficial, healing effect upon the body. You may use many of the relaxation techniques and pratyahara kriyas to develop this awareness.

The third stage is awareness of the mind and how the mind can control the emotions and the body. Adhi-Vyadhi is the sanskirit term for all diseases. These originate in your mind and manifest in your body. It is the term for psychosomatics in modern medical science. It is interesting that modern medicine is finding the root causes of diseases stemming from stress, emotional or psychological issues. This concept is not new to Yoga; in fact it is thousands of years old. Many of the therapies used today are to be found in ancient Yoga scriptures.

When this phase is accomplished, a new awareness can be sought, one in which the conscious mind is transcended by a higher aspect of the mind called Buddhi (intellect). Dharana, concentration and Dhyana, meditation are used to produce this awareness.

The fourth stage is "awareness of awareness" described as Samadhi or Cosmic Consciousness. I heartily pray to my Guru Swami Gitanada Giri Gurumaharajji to give us strength and ability to attain this stage of Samadhi.

Meenakshi Devi Bhavanani adds the fifth awareness to this fourfold awareness of Swamiji. That is the awareness of how unaware are we. To begin to walk on the path of awareness we need motivation and this can be enhanced once we come to know and recognise our unawareness.

Now you need to inculcate that awareness. Try to be aware of work, movements, walking, resting, eating, and talking. During Hatha Yoga practice be aware of your movements, stretching and relaxation, twists, body organs effected, sensations and stimulations, etc.

Don't be afraid of your ego, dullness, negative thoughts and emotions. You need to transcend them to grow on the path of evolution. Watch out if any pain is there. Watch out if there is any stress or stain. Watch out if there is any sorrow or negative emotion. You may observe your breath; heartbeats, movement of the diaphragm with the breath, and try to keep the mind concentrated in the body.

Know your every thought and emotion. Whenever you have negative thought or emotion you may use the mental repetition of om shanti, om shanti (Om Peace). There may be arousal of some spiritual experiences during the quietness of mind and emotions.

Try to observe your sleep. If you have some sleep disorder you may use the yoga-nidra or relaxation exercise before going to sleep. If possible try to develop the awareness of your dreams. This will develop the insight required for higher yoga in you.

Try to recall your good memories and develop a positive attitude regarding your self image. Always feel self-satisfied with what you have done. Feel gratitude for what you have. In Geeta Lord Krishna says that you do your duties and don't be worried for the fruits. Simply we conclude with the thought- "do your best and leave the rest."

Yoga as a holistic concept.

Yoga is the science of the whole of mankind. Yoga is also a spiritual path whose aim is individual realization in consciousness of the independent self-existing, self-originating, indwelling spirit of mankind.

Yoga is a way of life where the principles and practices of Yoga are made as the foundation of the spiritual life and one lives Yoga – fearlessly, the Yoga Life!

Yoga is highly ethical and intellectual. Yoga offers a safe method of concentration and meditation, educating practical application of the powers of the human mind. Yoga in its Kriyas and Prakriyas, methods and techniques deals with the government of the mind and the control and regulation of the emotions and the body by the Atman, the indwelling self. Its entire process is centred on awareness.

Does living the yoga path mean you don't have 'fun' anymore?

No, of course not! To some the outer appearance of a disciplined yoga life may appear so, but once you are firmly on the yoga path it is not so in your heart, quite the opposite. Once we have refined and balanced our energies, mental and emotional layers, we need very little to feel happiness. You will not need to experience extremes to feel something!

Yoga is the control of thought-waves in the mind that are achieved by means of practice and non-attachment. Practice becomes firmly grounded when it is cultivated for a long time, uninterruptedly, with earnest devotion. Non-attachment is the exercise of discrimination that may come very slowly. But even its earliest stages are rewarded by a new sense of freedom and peace. It should never be thought of as an austerity, a kind of self-torture, something grim and painful. The practice of non-attachment gives value and significance to even the most ordinary incidents of the dullest day. It eliminates boredom from our lives. As we progress and gain increasing self-mastery, we shall see that we are renouncing nothing that we really need or want, we are only freeing ourselves from imaginary needs and desires. In this spirit, a soul grows in greatness until it can accept life's worst disasters, calm and unmoved.

Yamas - Restraints

A strong building can only be built up on a strong foundation. If your foundation is weak, your building will collapse very soon. The same rule is applicable to the yogic approach of spiritual evolution. If your base of moral character, behaviour, attitude, thoughts, beliefs, emotions and finally physical actions are not right or correct, you can not grow on the path of yogic evolution. These days most of the modern yogic teachings avoid the importance of Yamas and Niyamas. In ancient times in India, you must have perfected these to some degree before you were allowed to study under a Yoga Master.

Swamiji Dr. Gitananda Giri Gurumaharajaji says that yamas and niyamas are the basic foundations of yogic evolution. Without perfecting them one cannot attain the highest stage of purity, bliss and joy. Yamas and niyamas are not optional in yoga; their perfection is not only needed but is essential for all yoga sadhakas (truth seekers).

In a yogic perspective, yama/niyama are not ends or goals in themselves, nor are they rules nor prescriptions, but merely remedial processes designed to help us to grow on the path of evolution of the inner eternal law (Sanatana Dharma).

Yamas are restraining our animal nature and then through the Niyamas we change lower energy to the higher energy of love, compassion, and respect for all.

In Hinduism 'Yama' is also known as the lord of death and death is unavoidable for all the living beings. Thus yamas should be followed and perfected like the ultimate goal of the life and one can attain the highest stage of yogic evolution only through perfection of the yamas and niyamas. One may break down the word, yama, in an unconventional way; 'ya' meaning that which moves, while 'ma' represents the mother principle: nature's/creation's nurturing principle. Thus in this analysis yama means to bring forth, nurture and move with the natural processes of creation. Death is an unavoidable truth of your birth.

The five Yamas are:
Ahimsa-satya-asteya-brahmacarya-aparigraha yamah. (Yoga-sutra. II 30.)

1. **Ahimsa** non-violence, i.e. the removal of violence from our own life as well as others taken in the non-dual sense, or that we are all one. This also includes protecting our own body and personal space from harm.
2. **Satya** truthfulness being the removal of the veils of deceit and falsehood from our lives including that of self deception.
3. **Asteya** honesty, non-stealing, non-exploitation of others, and integrity in all our relations.
4. **Brahmacharya** continuity, centeredness, wedded-ness, or one-pointedness to the all inclusive weave of "Source" - harmony and union in true Integrity while not allowing oneself to be distracted from the spiritual goal. Control of our ????? energy.

5. **Aparigraha** non-possessiveness, non-greed, non-envy, non-attachment, letting go, non-false identification penetrating throughout the mind in meditation as well as in all our relationships as the simplification of our life so that we are better able to focus on the spiritual goal latent in every moment.

Each Yama and Niyama could fill a book individually, but for a little insight I have expanded more. Yamas and Niyamas all have their root in ahimsa (not harming living beings); their aim is to perfect this love that we ought to have for all creatures.

Ahimsa, or non-violence is not harming or supporting any harmful activity to any one or the self through our thoughts, emotions and actions. Since everybody on the planet has caused some harm to other animal forms or plants, the spiritual truth that ahimsa points to is simply to more deeply commune and inter-connect with the practices of non-violence, not harming others or self, and actually removing harm to others (healing) and self especially in the transpersonal sense where "the other" and the self are one in our daily actions so that balance and continuity in our authentic yoga practice is accelerated and realised.

Satya or truth is being adhered to the truth and reality in all situations. Satya is also behaving righteously to save and protect the dharmas and humanity. In the yogic aspect satya is also to teach and speak about the yogic approaches and spirituality you have experienced and not by listening or reading from books.

It is not so concerned with "telling the truth" externally as much as it is in its inner (antar) esoteric meaning of removing the ingrained Samskaras which support self deceit and conceit.

In simple definition Samskaras are deep imprinted positive values of life in your personality. While in yogic perspective these are bondages of your positive and negative karmas/deeds in present and previous lives. To grow up on this spiritual path you have to work out all of them and there is no shortcut in the yoga path.

Thus satya should be practiced with the body, speech, and mind. Satya thus does not mean to restrain deceit as much as to bring forth Truth; i.e., to remove falsehood, confusion, illusion, delusion, and ignorance.

Brahmachariya as merely the sexual restraint is a misunderstanding of its practice and great values. Brahmachariya in its vast meanings is to adhere with the natural laws or the universal laws of this creation of Brahma. Brahmacharya is to reveal, acknowledge, and act in accordance with the eternal inner eternal teacher. Brahmacharya is practiced thus not as a restraint of the body, but within the integration of the body, speech, and mind as an affirmation of a way of life.

Asteya is not only non-stealing of material things, but also includes time, peace, privacy, and even thoughts. It is being honest in all aspects of individual as well as social life. Positive attitude, gratitude and being grateful to your parents, friends, and teachers for helping you or providing all these resources and knowledge are part of practising Asteya. On universal level caring for nature and not exploiting mother earth's resources is Asteya.

Aparigraha is not only to eliminate exploitation, contradiction, deceit, self dishonesty, greed, attachment, and selfishness, but to act to promote integrity, honesty, generosity, trust, abundance, fulfilment, and gratefulness, contentment, and clarity in body, mind and speech. Aparigraha is living your life with the minimum resources you need to live a healthy and happy life rather than accumulating everything even if you don't need them and can be used by others. This can help us to save the planet from environmental catastrophe.

Yamas - Beyond All Limitations

Jati-desa-kala-samaya-anavacchinnah sarva-bhauma maha-vratam (yoga-sutra. II 31.)
The above sutra means : adhering to these Yamas in all situations, at all times, without limitations or exceptions will turn the tide effecting closure of and sealing off the great gate of death and dissolution, thus moving us into greater synchronization with the natural laws of the universe as it is (Sanatana Dharma).

This sutra emphasizes on practice of all the yamas in each and every situation and not only with certain people or in certain situations. Yamas should be perfected with all the living races, in all the places and states, and at all times.

One can attain the highest stage only by perfecting the yamas, only then can we attain freedom from the cycle of life and death. Practicing yamas with body, mind and emotions with each and every situation is the way of cleansing out your past karmas and bondages of the karmas.

It is seen that the root of all the sins is the bhaya, or fear and clinging to life of the survival instincts at any cost (abhivinasha). Thus one should try to develop detachment, as in Lord Krishna's teaching in the Geeta that "you do your duty without desiring for the fruits." Swami Vivekananda also emphasized that to develop all the humane values you need to be fearless. So be fearless! Be fearless!

Thus yamas are to protect the inner as well as outer self, or real self which is a part of Mother Nature. These should be perfected in reference of human beings, animals, plants and the environment. If you are damaging the real or true form of nature, this is violence or untruthful behaviour for our upcoming generations.

Niyamas- Duties to be Adhered to for Evolution

'Ni', means that which is inherent or underneath. As such the niyamas clarify, complement, and expand upon the yamas. The niyamas thus are even more proactive actions that Patanjali encourages us to undertake in order to accelerate one's success in yoga. Yama and niyama are both leading to the same destination. For example, ahimsa and satya promote saucha and swadhyaya, asteya and aparigraha lead to santosha and tapas, brahmacharya leads to isvara pranidhana, while the reverse is also true; i.e., that the practice of the niyama leads to the realization of the yamas.

After restraining the animal instincts by perfecting the yamas you come to the point of building up human nature and this starts with the practice of the niyamas in yoga. All animal instincts are inborn characteristics in all of us. The human nature has to be encouraged in us. This work starts with the teachings in family by our parents, grandparents, relatives, society and school. They teach us naturally how to behave with our body, mind and emotions and then how to behave properly with others in different situations. So if you will do swadhyaya you will find that the foundation of all the yamas is being made from the first day of your life you started to learn.

1. Saucha on a gross physical level is the obvious general cleanliness of the body and appearance as well as abstaining from poisoning the body or burdening it with food and drinks that it can not be digested, assimilated, or eliminated easily. This will unburden not only the digestive system, but the elimination and immune systems thus creating more available energy for the process of evolutionary higher consciousness to unfold. Another inner application of Saucha is keeping the manomaya kosha (mental thoughts / energy body) free from all the negativities. So in normal life keeping your body, mind, emotions on individual level and then cloths, surroundings, and environment on external level is Saucha.

Saucha may be applied to our belief systems whether or not they may be tainted, and thus be a source of taint, impurity, and affliction to our consciousness (until purified). In this sense transformation and rebirth is an action of purification. Yet another manifestation of Saucha is in our motivations and actions. But since actions follow thought and consciousness (or lack thereof) it seems that the purification of consciousness is more significant to this process.

2. Santosha is contentment, fulfilment, completion, and peace. As such it denotes abundance (not scarcity), happiness (not discontent), and in a deeper sense especially deep gratitude. By gratitude, one does not need to be grateful to any person or event, but rather it is the deep heartily felt sense of unconditional gratitude.
Santosha is practiced as peace and happiness as love. We commune with peace and abundance and give it forth- manifest it. When greed, lust, conflict, war, trickery, competition, himsa (violence), pain, thievery, deceit, corruption, falsity, and ignorance are defeated; when the invincible Supreme Self is victorious; then Santosha reigns supreme! In the meanwhile we must attempt to assess our allegiance with grief, war, conflict, anger, hatred, jealousy, hurt, and fear; be willing to surrender them and to alter them to peace and lasting happiness.

'Kriya yoga'... Niyamas continued

Patanjali states that one can directly attain the samadhi or oneness only through perfecting the three niyamas- tapas, swadhyaya and isvar-pranidhan. These three together are also termed as kriya-yoga (this does not refer to the Kriya Yoga of Paramhansa Yogananada).

3. Tapas is not simply renunciation, but rather a recycling of the energy that could have been placed into further distraction and dissipation; placing this energy into one's spiritual evolution. Tapas becomes the activity that freshens up and sparks a practice that has become sluggish and dull. As such then it is an affirmation of the higher Self. This is the action of authentic tapas. Very simply by letting go of one's attachment in such neurotic activities or propensities, then space and energy is liberated and reclaimed that can now be directed toward pure essence or supreme self.

4. Swadhyaya is not merely "scriptural study" or book study. Although studying "right spiritual" philosophy and practicing contemplation on mental and psychological phenomena (jnana yoga) can provide some specific benefits of clarification or insight to higher aspects. Such external study can be often very misleading and disorientating (unless balanced with inner study).

Thus in a yogic sense swadhyaya means studying, observing, and eventually knowing our true self nature, not through the conceptual confines and objective externalized eyes of the intellect, books, scripture, or authority, but rather through Gnosis acquired through meditation; from an authentic direct transpersonal experience. This study or inquiry into Self is an essential practice of the process of self realisation via the removal of delusion/illusion (maya).

5. Isvara is often mistranslated with the English term, "God", which in the Western sense of the term, is almost the opposite of what is meant because Isvara specifically is not a theistic idea (as yoga is not theistic). In other words the word Isvara specifically refers to the formless and deity-less, "aspectless aspect" of the divine aspect of Reality in Yoga. Thus Isvara pranidhana is to surrender to the great integrity of formless infinity which is the eternal (beginning-less and ending-less). The word, Isvara, thus expresses or symbolizes completeness, the whole or infinite mind and as

such cannot be represented by symbols being the nothingness that includes everything.
The following four verses of yoga sutras clarify all the misleading thoughts regarding the Isvara-

Klesha-karma-vipakasayair apara-mrshta purusa-visesa isvarah (Sutra 24)- Isvara is the purest (a-para-mrshta) aspect (visesa) of pure undifferentiated universal consciousness (purusa) which is untouched and unaffected by taint (klesha), karma, and the seed germs (asayair) that result (vipaka) from ordinary desire and propensities.

Tatra-nir-atishayam sarvajna-bijam(Sutra 25) -There (tatra) [isvara] is the seed and origin (bija) of absolute (nir-atishayam), unsurpassed, and complete omniscience (sarvajna).

Tasya vachakah pranavah(Sutra 27) - Isvara is expressed and represented (vachakah) by the vibratory energy contained in the pranava (the sacred syllable, om).

Taj-japas tad-artha-bhavanam(Sutra 28) - Through generating (bhavanam) constant repetition (taj-japa) of the pranava (om) the meaning (artha) behind the sound is realised and becomes manifest (bhavanam).

In the "Geeta" Lord Krishna says: "Many are the means described for the attainment of the highest goal....but love is the highest of all; love and devotion that make one forget everything else; love that merge the devote with me...as all earthly pleasure fade into nothingness." The path of love is considered supreme because it is wholly selfless and eternal the total erasing of self for the love of the Supreme Self. The chains of desire bind us. The Jnani's strength and knowledge breaks the chains; the Bhakta, on the other hand, becomes so small and ego-less they slip through the chains. In bhakti, the mind melts in love for God and so is dissolved in Supreme Soul. In Jnana, the mind is mastered and over-powered by the force of wisdom. The same is described in the following three verses of the yoga sutras:
Samadhi-siddhir Isvara-pranidhanat(II 45.)-Samadhi is perfected (siddhir) through letting go the limited matrix of a separate self while surrendering to isvara (the all inclusive aspectless and unconditioned great universal integrity

or the underlying motive power behind the principle of Infinite Mind).

Sauca-samtosa-tapah-svadhyaya-isvara-pranidhanani niyamah (II 32.) - Niyama consists of saucha (purity), santosha (contentment and peacefulness), tapas (spiritual passion and fire), swadhyaya (self study and mastery), and Isvara pranidhana (surrender to the Universal Great Integrity of Being).

Tapah-svadhyayesvara-pranidhanani kriya-yogah(II.1) - Tapas (spiritual passion, energy, or heat generated through forgoing dissipative activities), swadhyaya (self study), and isvara pranidhana (the function of surrender to or the embrace of the all encompassing comprehensive integrity which interconnects us all (who we really are) are the three essential prerequisite (kriya) activities that lead us to realizing the fruit of yoga.

Sri Sathya Sai Baba says; "love is the most powerful thing in the world…. All the yogas are included in the path of the love, and whoever attains this love, attains God."

Mystics and Saints of all religions have testified the beauty of supreme love. 'It is the power that makes the sun and stars to move' said Dante. According to scriptures, God created this universe for love and that love is the very purpose of our existence. Love confirms Ananda/Bliss and softens the grind of mundane existence.

Tyagraj sang: "Is there greater Bliss O God, than to dance, to sing to you, to pray for your presence, and unite with you in my mind?" The Narada Bhakti Sutras describe Bhakti as a transcendental experience of bliss, in which the ego is completely dissolved and absorbed, in the Supreme Soul.

Love is without boundaries and ever expanding, like God, who is limitless. The love of Gopis (lovers) for Krishna is celebrated in our scriptures because of its glorious nature. Such love transcends mind and the body and touches the soul.

Divine love is free from any motive. Divine love is transitory, a pure reflection of the real thing. Worldly love is erratic and subject to change; but love for God is unchanging and eternal, everlasting. Divine love is perfect, it is always charged with its own energy. It is nitya- nautnam or fruitful and ever new.

To attain this state, however, we have to pay a price. Meera Bai, 16th century Saint-Poet, sang: "Kanha, the price He asked, I gave. Some cry, I gave in full, weighed to the utmost grain, my love, my life, my soul, my all...." As mystics have testified there is peace and fulfilment in devotion that nothing else can bring.

A devotional prayer with total devotion for the supreme self.

> "I pray not for wealth,
> I pray not for ownership,
> I pray not for pleasures or even for the joys of poetry.
> I only pray that during all my life,
> I may have love:
> That I may have love to God

The incorporation of these yamas / niyamas into our daily lives will serve as guideposts to show us where we go astray and where we can better connect more completely and continuously with the Source. These guidelines of ahimsa, truthfulness, integrity, non-possessiveness, continuity, purity, peacefulness, divine passion, self study, and surrender can also be expediently applied to our daily asana practice to accelerate to its highest accomplishment as well.

Hatha-Yoga Concept and Benefits of Asanas

Hatha yoga and all the Tantric practices are based on the concept of the loma-viloma. The Sanskrita word 'hatha' is derived from the joining of 'ha' and 'tha'. 'Ha' is the solar energy represented by the warm golden sun. 'Tha' is the lunar energy represented by the cool silvery moon. The aim of all the hatha yoga and tantric practices is union and balancing of the 'ha' and 'tha'; solar and lunar energies, within the body.

Our half right part of body is represented by the masculine characters of shiva and left half body is representation of the feminine characters of shakti. This sun and moon; warm golden and cool silvery; ha and tha; energies are known as loma and viloma respectively. These are also represented by the prana and apana energies.

Prana moves from the top to the bottom in the right half of the body whilestapana moves from the bottom to the top in the left half of the body. This is also found in the concept of the polarity of the human body. Energy always flows in the wide oval shape in and out side the body.

Our human life is a representation of five bodies, or panch-koshas. These are annamaya kosha, or the physical body; pranamaya kosha or the psychic body; manomaya kosha or the mental body; anadamaya kosha or the blissful body; vijnanamaya kosha or the pure subtle body or the soul. The loma and viloma energies are manifestation of the positive energy and the negative energy from the subtle to the gross body.

The process of human evolution from the animal nature to the human nature and then to the purest nature of super conscious is from the gross or the physical body. Body awareness and awareness of the loma and viloma energies refines and purify these energies to their subtle forms to gain the harmony and oneness with the self and nature.

The five gross pranas, apana, vyana, prana, samana and udana flow in various parts of our body in various directions to keep the physical, mental and emotional process in health and harmonious functioning. They regulate the normal functioning of the body area they are concerned with.

Asanas are designed to align the body skeletal system. These strengthen the legs, thighs, pelvic area muscles, and shoulders.

Asanas reduce the fat of the hips, thighs, and abdomen and west region. These are also good for directing the blood flow to the inner parts of the knees, thighs, and lower back region and thus eradicate the toxins accumulated there.

It directs the blood flow towards the heart and lungs and thus prevents the chances to develop any of the coronary and heart diseases. All sections of lungs are activated and reproduced. They also provide a very good message to the digestive organs and increase the digestive fire.

Postures are also of high importance in the spiritual aspects as most of the shapes of the asanas are related to our psychic energy centres, charkas, e.g. triangle shape / Trikanasana.

Asanas also reverse the blood flow and pranic energy in the body. They also generate the sensitivity and awareness of the whole body muscles and organs and thus are of great importance to practice concentration and especially shavasana (yogic relaxation pose) and the yoga-nidra. Shavasana and yoga-nidra are pre-requisite for meditation.

Asanas are aimed to align the body skeletal system. Whole body joints are loosened and this increases their mobility. Bones are strengthened and their rigidity is removed. This prevents the bone decomposition and thus keeps us fit until old age. Asanas contain various forward and back stretching positions which help to balance our energies;
The silvery cool apana moves from bottom to the top of the body. This is also known as shakti or the feminine energy in all human beings. Prana moves from the top of the body to the bottom. This golden prana is also known as shiva, or masculine energy.

According to Maharishi Patanjali, "sthiram sukham asanam" which means a firm, and comfortable position is asana or posture. Here Maharshi states that a firm and pleasing position in which sadhaka can sit for higher spiritual practices is known as asana.

In the Bhagavad-Gita Lord Krishna states that a sadhaka in asana should sit with an erect spine neck and head then gaze constantly at the tip of the nose and contemplate ME (God).

According to Shiva-samahita there are 84 million postures and asanas which are associated with the yoni or creation or different species. Many asanas presently are associated with birds and animals such as matsyasana (fish posture), mayurasana (peacock posture), bakasana (herring), mandukasana (frog), etc.

In authentic scriptures of Hatha-yoga 32 asanas are mentioned. Four of them are most important – Sukkha asana (pleasant pose), Padma asana (lotus pose), Varjra asana (thunderbolt pose), Siddha asana (perfect pose).

Presently the meaning of asanas is changed and expanded. Now asanas are used for strength, stamina and health promotion. Normally yoga is considered as merely a few asanas and pranayamas. Asanas are often performed in acrobatic style to maintain slim and beautiful body.

In ancient times asanas were practiced for transforming the lower sexual energy in to higher spiritual energy. It was aimed to balance the pancha-koshas, pancha-pranas and shiva-shakti or loma-viloma energy aspects.

The aim of all yogic practices is unity of both the feminine and masculine energies in our body to attain the oneness or union of the self with the supreme self. Asanas have a complete approach to transverse the apana and prana in the middle anahata chakra for the union or merging in each other. It refines the gross prana to the subtle pure prana, which is essential to realize the higher aspects of yogic practices.

Pranayama

Pranayama yoga is the "science of breath", the control of the vital force (prana) present in the air we breath. The Sanskrita term pranayama means: 'Prana' is the divine universal creative energy or power, and the 'yama' means control or the science of control.

The word 'prana' can be broken further as 'pra' means to exist independently, or to have the prior existence. 'Ana' is shortened term of 'anna' means a cell, or collectively 'ana'. Thus 'prana' means "that which existed before any atomic or the cellular life came into being". Such life is termed as manifestation of the divine.

Behind all the manifestation of creation and life is this divine energy prana. Most of the prana we receive from the air we inhale. But we also receive it to some extent from water and food. Some part is also absorbed directly in the skin from the atmosphere.

Remember that the prana is not oxygen or the other gases we inhale nor the nutrients we take from the food. The truth is that behind using all these nutrients and the gases for breathing this divine energy prana plays the role as the catalyst. Prana is absorbed through the exposed nerve endings of the body and especially in the nostrils, mouth and back of the throat. Thus eat slowly and chew properly to allow the releasing and absorbing of the prana. Water should be sipped slowly to allow the absorption of prana in the throat and mouth.

We must learn pranayama from the beginning to do Dirgha Pranayama, deep slow and controlled breath. Most of us nowadays are shallow breathers and lacking the prana or the oxygen for the normal functioning of our body, mind and emotions. Most of the present diseases are because of improper breathing. All illnesses can be alleviated by practicing pranayama properly and by attaining perfection in them. For a yogi the breathing should be under the total awareness. This conscious breathing brings the autonomic functions under the control of the nervous system or the will.

Improper breathing, dyspnoea or laboured breathing is not a recent problem. But now it becomes more prominent because of a stressful lifestyles and the adverse environmental conditions making it worse. Even Yogi Gorakshanatha travelled the whole of the India and gave the message-

"O men and women of India! You have defaulted from the good health by being the shallow breathers".

He stated that in his age people were breathing only one-eight of their capacity. He cured many of the diseases only by teaching the asanas and pranayamas.

When we do shallow breathing, the nerve receptors sited deep in the lungs are unaffected. Only when we breathe in and out deeply these inspiratory and expiratory receptors get stimulated and called for their desired activity. This sends the reflexo-genic feed-back to the brain. This governs the control over the in and out breath along with the hold in and hold the out breath.

Breath is also related to our life and spirit or the soul. Even it is said that there is life in the body, if there is breath in the body. In Sanskrita word Brahman is used for the breath. In taking the breath is termed as inspiration in Greek, which comes from 'in-spiro' means being in tune with the spirit or the God. While expiration is originated from the 'ex-piro' means to be out of the spirit. In India if some one dies they say in Hindi 'prana tyaga diye' which means literally that 'prana left the body'.

The yogis performed the pranayamas and found that they can fulfil their need of prana only through the air with no other sustenance. They don't need to eat food and are known as breatharians. Still there are yogis in various parts of the world those who are alive without food and even some are without water.

Pranayama is Not only a Breathing Exercise

Simply a yogic practice called pranayama where one starts by first taking firm and pleasant asana (sthirama-sukham-asanam), then turning attention upon the inhalation and exhalation of the breath in order to extend and refine (ayama) the prana. According to Patanjali **Pranayama is an awareness/ observation practice, not a mechanical practice.**

First you all should know that the most common mistranslation- "pranayama is the control or regulation of the inhalation, exhalation, and retention of breath". Then in this case we should call it 'swashayama'.

The first misinterpretation of the word, prana, as breath, which makes the definition redundant as well as misleading. Pranayama is the extension, spreading, thinning, refinement, or expansion of energy, where prana is life energy and "ayama" is expansion, thinning, rarefaction, or extension.

The definition of yama as control or regulation, reflects concepts of hatha yoga which believed that liberation could be attained through forcefulness and control of the body, breath, and mind. Similar mistranslations: nirodha as control, tapas as self abnegation, swadhyaya as scriptural study, or brahmacharya as sexual restraint where there exists no objective or experiential basis.

We have to learn to expand and refine the prana by observing and breaking apart the movements of the breath as it occurs in inspiration and expiration so that it is no longer controlled by the unconscious winds of karma, thoughts, emotions and unconscious habits, but rather it comes into the light of awareness. In this way our energy and mind changes as well as our karma.

Pranayama can be started first as the process (gati) of becoming aware of our vital energy by breaking it down into its gross external components as manifest in the profound linkages between mind and energy inherent in the breathing process. Try to inculcate the awareness of how the energy enters our body/mind, how it leaves it, and how it becomes discontinuous or inhibited. Then we obtain awareness of how the energy is extended, refined, and made more subtle so that we open up the nadis (the flows of the prana) which activates the body's higher potential.

Prana (with a capital "P" permeates all of the Universe without it nothing moves, but also prana with a small "p" denotes the vital energy (prana) as it permeates the physical body. It is strongly associated with the breath as the animating principle- as the sustained-linking creation with Infinite Source.
Indeed breathing is the most primal activity of human life. Breath performs a bridge between the unconscious (autonomic) and conscious (central) nervous systems. In hatha. kundalini, and tantra yoga pranayama is not just a powerful awareness tool, but a focused practice capable of balancing and synchronizing not only the autonomic and central nervous systems, but also the afferent and efferent nervous systems and the sympathetic and parasympathetic nervous systems as all polarities can be accessed through the breath. Similarly, hatha yoga tells us that by becoming aware of and accessing the breath consciously in these ways we can also access directly into our **psycho-neurology**, the biopsychic pathways, nadis, matrices, energy cysts, and cellular and energetic imprints which hold the samskaras in place, thus breaking them up, breaking up past karma, kleshas, and vrttis (root desires).

Thus the various pranayama exercises of exploring the energetic processes of inhalation, exhalation, and ?????? of breath especially in Gitananda Rishiculture Yoga were given to Sadakas in order to achieve this awareness, observe this process, and thus eventually achieve purity of body, mind and emotions followed by karmic purification to attain liberation (from karma and vrtti). The goal is not the control of the breath. Our goal is to inculcate the awareness of the subtle and eternal operations of prana shakti or kundalini shakti.

In many practices of hatha yoga, laya yoga, and prana vidya, control of the normal flow of the breath are given in order to both develop awareness and oneness. The Second aim is to disrupt old mental patterns (vrttis) and karma fructifying the previous dormant or energy to spiritual evolution. These innumerable pranayama practices one has the opportunity to investigate many types of breathing patterns upon on our energy field and thus becoming aware of the breath processes (vicchedah), then one becomes more aware and integrated with Vital Prana.

"Normal" subconscious habitual breathing is thus called karmic breathing, while pranayama practice not only breaks up old karma, but burns it up to make practitioner free of karmic bondage. Here various pranayama practices using the breath can be used for healing, and propelling the practitioner beyond their past conditioning and karma altogether. Just simple breath awareness helps us to free the dissipations of the 'monkey-like' mind (vikalpa) and concentrates the chi-prana. In Rishiculture tradition pranayama practices go deeper and work faster combining, pranayama, pratyhara, dharana, mudra, and asana as one integrated practice.

In simple pranayama like sukha-pranayama or the vibhhaga pranayama we can simply notice the changing qualities of breath according to how the mind becomes distracted or focused. We bring our awareness to the breath and refine and extend it if it has become coarse or restricted. After practice this relationship between the empty and quiet mind and the breath becomes harmonious and a doorway opens into the operations of the cit-prana and the operations of the mind. Then eventually the origin of mind, the Infinite Mind, or simply the Natural Unconditioned Mind is revealed through at first the very simple method learning how to observe the breath and how it changes. Then one learns how to balance and direct the cit-prana, the mind, and the breath all at once.

Pranayama brings us into awareness of the polar opposites, the expansion and the contraction of the divine pulsation of siva/shakti (spanda), the movement of spirit as it inspires, and eternal dance of love through the expiratory medium of the living temple.

Basic Requirements for Good Pranayama

First if you have any of the breathing problems related to shallow breathing that should be corrected. Then the environmental conditions should be also considered to be free from dust or a damp atmosphere. Proper sectional breathing should be practiced. Your mat should be of thin and firm, like a rubber-foam pad. A thick mattress stuffed with the cotton and other softeners tends to catch the dust, and germs detrimental to the correct breathing.

Your room should be regularly cleaned. Never allow the dirt to accumulate on the walls, corners, and other cloths you are using. Bed covers and other cloths should be of cotton.

Use of the powders, fumes, scents, essences, body lotions etc should be avoided and especially in case you have any allergic problems. Even you may be allergic to the soap, tooth powder, or the facial creams, be aware and avoid the harmful things.

The preparation should be done properly before starting the pranayama or the hatha yoga practice, ideal conditions are:

- Comb and tie up your hair properly. Loose hair may create problems in complete breathing.

- Clean your body before the practice by light warm bath. Please never take too hot too cool bath before the hatha yoga practice.

- Clean, loose comfortable clothes should be worn if possible. Tight clothes, jewellery, belts, etc should be avoided.

- After the yoga practice a cool shower should be taken. This will strengthens the body tolerance power to cold air and water. Although this will depend on where you live in the world!

- Keep your mat properly folded and covered with the cotton cloths to avoid the damp and dust.

- Your area of practicing yoga should be well-ventilated with plenty of fresh air.

- Do all the practice at least after three hours of eating the food. All practices should be done with an empty stomach. A light tea, lemon or limewater can be taken. Avoid all the mucus producing foods. If there is any desire to empty the bowel or bladder, do so, as a priority.

Prana, Thoughts and Emotions

Try to remember the situation when you are very happy and cheerful; how do you feel about your body and about your self at that time? You feel very light, energetic, and willing to do everything at that moment. What is behind all this?

Now remember the situation when you are sad, unhappy and in bad mood; how do you feel about your body and yourself? You feel very heavy, tired, exhausted, lack of interest and will. What is behind all this?

As we have discussed that all of our physical, mental and emotional process are carried on through the energy of prana. So our mental and emotional states directly affect the levels of prana in us. All the negative thoughts, stress and negative emotions blocks the refinement of prana and flow of the prana in the naris (also known as nadis, energy channels in the body). They consume a high amount of the prana because the negative thoughts create the body reactions of an 'emergency state'. Our autonomic nervous system and the endocrine nervous system have to prepare for the fight-flight response. This consumes a lot of prana and preparation for nothing. So be careful about what you think and feel.

Patanjali describes that in all the adverse mental and emotional processes use the opposite thought or the emotion to get rid of the negativity (pratipaksha-bhavanam).

It is also stated in the Upanishadas that your prana goes; where your awareness goes. So the more distracted your thoughts and emotions are, the more your prana is scattered or poor. Paradoxically, the more refined your awareness is the greater your power to manifest your thoughts.

In the Bhagavad-Gita Lord Krishna states that the mind is the vehicle of prana. Thus your awareness goes where your thought goes. Your mind goes where your awareness goes and there goes the prana. Thus the mind or the thoughts and emotions need the prana or the consciousness to travel in and out. Those who do mental work at the end of the day feel more tired in comparison to the person doing only physical work, why? Our mental and emotional processes consume more prana than the physical process. So be careful and aware of what you think and what you feel, develop your awareness of the mental and emotional processes.

Prana- Philosophical Aspect

According to Indian schools of philosophies, i.e. Upanishads, Samkhya, Advaita, etc., the body is divided in two parts – the gross physical body (sthul sarira) and the subtle body (linga sarira), both include five Pranas, the mind (mental body), the intellectual (buddhi) and the self-sense (ahankara). The gross physical body in composed of five elements. According to Nyaya philosophy the body is the vehicle of action for the self. The mind along with all sense organs is found to operate only within the human body. All feelings of pleasure and pain in the body are due the destiny (karma). Balanced functioning of sympathetic and parasympathetic parts of the nervous system is necessary for the harmony in all these, described above.
The Indian yogis described the energy of Prana, as the vital energy essential for a living being. According to some of the six Indian philosophies "Prana is a subtle life-force". Some times it is represented as an electromagnetic force or bioelectric force in the body, but not exactly these can be described as the Prana, though these are similar to the Prana. The term Prana is more appropriate to describe the Prana as the vital life force.

Prana sustains and supports this body. All the bodily activities are dependent of the pranic energy. According to Indian Yoga, "When the Queen bee goes up all the Bees go up, and as the Queen Bee settles down all the Bees settle down, when so, speech, mind, sense are balanced when the energy of Prana is balanced in human body.

According to the six schools of Indian philosophies, everything in this universe is composed of cosmic energy, Prana. In various schools, like Vedic, Samkhya, Jain etc., the Prana is classified in five categories, which flow in various parts of the body and regulates their concerned functions. In upanishadas and other tantric yogic texts five up-pranas are also stated and detailed.

Pancha Vayus

Vayu	Body Region	Movement	Area Between	Function
1. Prana	heart region	Upward	larynx and diaphragm	breathing, food and liquid swallowing
2. Apana	lower regions	Downward	Navel and perineum	Elimination of urine, faeces, gas, wind, sexual fluids, menstrual blood, and the foetus at the time of birth
3. Samana	Digestive area	Lateral moving	Diaphragm and navel	All digestive functions and also the heating and cooling of the body
4. Udana	Peripheral parts	Spiraling	Above the larynx and also the arms	Brain and all sensory receptors- eyes, ears, nose, tongue and skin are governed as well as three organs of action-speech, hands and feet
5. Vyana	All-pervasive	All directions	Whole body	Reserve force for all four and maintenance of their depletion, regulation of physical movements

Pancha Upa-Prana Vayus

Upa-prana	Function
Naga	Belching, vomiting or spitting
Korma	Flickering of the eyes
Krikariya	Sneezing
Devadatta	Yawning
Dhananjaya	Physical warmth and remain in body for some time even after death

For controlling the senses, thoughts and emotions, it is not enough to acknowledge the anatomy and physiology of the human body, but also to be familiar with the flow of Prana. Hence for spiritual masteries, it is necessary to perceive the body as a whole. The process of body perception is the process of regulation of the prana in the body and development of detachment with that of the outer world and attachment with internal world. Hence it is the process of introversion and awakening of spiritualism.

Naris and Pranayama

The yoga science describes 72000 nadis; important among these are six, Ida, pingla, sushumna, brahmani, chitrani and vijnana. Most important are pingla (surya), which flow through right nostril; ida (Chandra), which flow through left nostril; sushumna (central) that is a movement when both nostrils flow freely without any obstruction.

Nari | **Body Part**
1. Ida Nari- | Left Side of Body
2. Pingala Nari | Right side of body
3. Shusumna Nari | Middle of body
4. Gandhari | left eye
5. Hastajiva | right eye
6. Pusha | right ear
7. Yashasavini | left ear
8. Alambusa | Facial region
9. Kuhu | Genitals
10. Shakini | Perineum

All these major nadis originate at the base of spine and travel upwards. The sushumna nadi is centrally located and travel along the spinal cord. At the level of larynx it divides into an anterior portion and a posterior portion, both of which terminate in the brahmarandra, or in cavity of Brahma. The ida and pingla also travel upwards along the spinal column, but they criss-cross the sushumna, before terminating in the left and right nostrils.

The junctions of the ida, the pingla, and the sushumna are known as charkas or wheels. There are seven principle chakras according to various Indian schools of yoga. These are: -

1. The muladhara chakra, (at the base of spine at the level of pelvic plexus).
2. The swadhishthana chakra (at the level of hypo gastric plexus).
3. The manipura chakra (at the level of solar plexus).
4. Anahata chakra (at the level of cardiac plexus).
5. The vishuddhia chakra (at the level of pharyngeal plexus).
6. The ajna chakra (at the level of nasoscilliary plexus).
7. The sahasrara chakra (at the top of head).

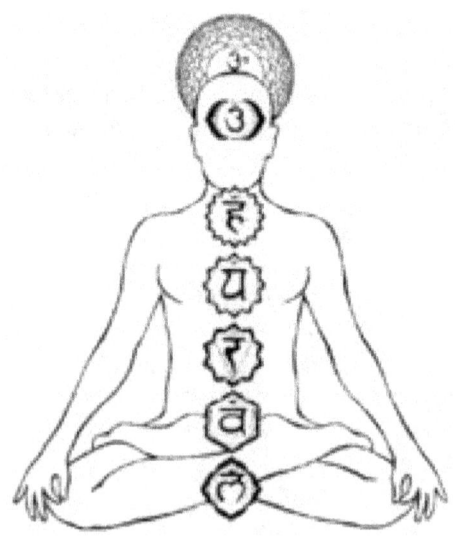

A fraction of the total energy of prana is used in dynamic and creative aspect; the major part of it is being in a potential, or seed state. The stored up energy is known as kundalini in manuals of yoga, the symbolic representation of which is that of a sleeping serpent rolled up in the muladhara charka, at the base of the spine. In the average individual there is flow of prana through the Ida and the pingla, but not through the sushumna, the nadi being blocked at the base of the spinal column.

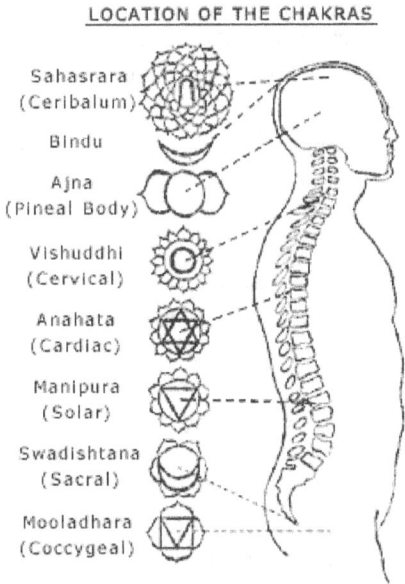

LOCATION OF THE CHAKRAS

Sahasrara (Ceribalum)
Bindu
Ajna (Pineal Body)
Vishuddhi (Cervical)
Anahata (Cardiac)
Manipura (Solar)
Swadishtana (Sacral)
Mooladhara (Coccygeal)

Pranayama is aimed to balance the ida and pingala nari to allow the free flow of the prana in the sushumna nari to attain the unity or the oneness with the supreme self. Pranayama opens all the blockages created because of our unhealthy life style and bad karmas. Pranayama refines and purifies the gross prana to the subtle and pure chitta-prana which enables us to feel the joy of oneness or samadhi the highest stage of yoga. This purification is a must for all the yogic seekers if you really want to grow on the path of yogic evolution. You have to purify your body, thoughts, emotions, karmas, and then gross prana to the subtle prana.

How to Meditate

Human beings are going towards spiritual teachings in search of mental peace. Try to feel calm and relax by using the medicine of spiritual teachings.

Like a drug addiction, some 'spiritual' teachings are also one type of addiction. Some times this may be so deep that it may cause family disputes.

Distance is developed between husband and wife. This distance may be so long that it may result in the breaking of relations.

Spirituality always binds the person with the person. That is not spirituality, which cause disputes in us. Can you call it spirituality that forms a wall between two?

Tension cannot be released by the action based meditation techniques and the ways of addiction. The action-based means may result in forgetting the tension for some time but this could not make one free from the stress.

Tension is released by meditation, but people have changed the picture of meditation in to pictures of actions. In the classes of meditation various activities are introduced in the name of meditation.

Reactions cannot be changed by the reactions. Reactions can be changed by inaction. Meditation is not action but meditation is inaction.

Meenakshi Devi Bhavanani often said during her satsanga (at Ananda Ashram, Puducherry, India) that "meditation is concentrating more and more on less and less, finally this becomes nothing or one-ness with dharana, and that merging in the self is called meditation, one needs to be purified to tolerate this stage of meditation". One should be physically stable and balanced, mentally and emotionally pure and calm. The brain should be healthy to perceive the mind and emotions. The naris should be purified for free flow of the prana from the lower charkas to the higher. This could be attained through the practices of asanas, Pranayama, and cleansing techniques.

We are prisoners of the sense organs and have to work in the outer world, so sense control through pratyahara should be perfected. Even **Dr. Swami Gitananda Giri** states that "the perfection of yamas and niyamas is the pre-condition to grow on the yogic path and this is compulsory for one and all".

Speech and listening also influences your progress in the path of meditation. Condition your mind in such a way that you speak and listen to things promoting you towards enlightenment. Do not waste time in gossiping, and in agitating thoughts and activities. The Mind is led to dullness by regular opposition of the light of Viveka. This can be enlightened by the practice of reflection, concentration and spiritual enquiry.

One can attain relaxation and stillness of body and mind through meditation. How do we meditate? When you come to this point we need to understand that meditation is **'not doing'**, or keeping our mind busy in structured practices or full of imaginative visualisations. However, our mind is so conditioned with our experiences, language, culture etc... therefore we always misunderstand the actual meaning of meditation. Meditation is going beyond all our 'doings' i.e. Physical, mental and imaginative processes. For this level to be reached, one must practice and repeat many of the breathing and structured relaxation techniques in order to break our conditioning.

To attain this world we have to consider the body and mind. We cannot perform the worldly activities without means of actions. The word and action is necessary to be with this physical world. But if you want to go beyond this world than one should be free from word and action. The body travels to action and mind up to the words. We trained the body for activities and taught words to the mind.
At the time of the body's birth it was unaware of the action. The brain possesses no words. The brain was empty. In which environment the bodies grow, the brain learned the language of the concerned area. The child learns from family members. We teach her/him to do something with her/his hands etc.

The senses are trained like this as s/he grows. The senses have the natural powers to do the actions. The brain also has an inborn ability to learn words. Our nature is inborn 'animal like' and it will remain so unless we learn higher aspects in this or the next life...

In the field of duties, the body and mind are important; word and action are valuable. But we have to go to the field of meditation. This is not the field of body and mind but it is the field of conscious, which is out of the reach of body and mind.

The body is visible and soul is invisible. The world is visible and the supreme soul is invisible. Now you want to say that we always try to visualize but cannot perceive it. The body has the ability to do only activities.

When the individual feels tired after actions, the energy is consumed the activities are stopped and relaxed. The power of perception of each sense organ has limitations. After a limit all activities are stopped.

It is also true that the brain have many unlimited abilities. The bird of the mind can fly in the space of imagination. But each bird has its limitations. If it will fly away from its limits then it is going to fall down. If the vehicle of the mind runs faster than the limits, it may also be damaged. The excessive use of the mind or the excessive weight of the words on the mind results in the mental imbalances which manifest in physical problems.

To gain this success we have to learn to meditate. The balance should be established between the action and word. The music to balance the body and mind is to be learned.

To meditate we consider the body and mind to catch the thread of action and word. The use of word and action is useful for the travelling of the external physical world; we can go on the steps of physical development. The help of action and word should be left to travel the internal world. If we try to enter the internal world along with the thread of action and world, there will be an opposing conflict.

The body and mind are god-gifted vehicles. The travelling of humanity and service in the nature of God is to be started by using these vehicles. Vehicles (bodies) are very important to go outside the home and to come back to the door of your home. Do you enter in your personal room with your vehicle? You leave your vehicle at your home's gate and then enter into your home.

When the senses begin to rest inward, rather than being distracted outwardly, then it means the vehicle returns back to home from the visit. Now you have to leave the vehicle and go for the rest in your personal room for the deep rest. Your personal room is full of the essence of peace. There is joy everywhere in that room, it is termed supreme soul. It is always present there. This stage is attained by consciousness/awareness. But our awareness learned the travelling in the visible world along with the body and mind.

Sadguru taught that the practice of rest in self-room is inaction meditation, or not doing, going beyond doing. The vehicle returns back to home. Fatigue of body and mind is released. Tension is also released. Awareness is merged in self. Where the awareness always meets with the psyche, where there is wordless rest.

Yoga - Uniting the Self and Supreme Self

Yoga is the process of taking us back to our un-distracted true nature. Yoga is the process of being one with self and the supreme self. Yoga is aimed to refine and purify all our mental, emotional and karmic bondages.

The Yoga-Sutras define that stage of mental and emotional destruction as not natural but modified. These modifications and afflictions are called chitta-vrttis. The state, called chitta-vrtti, is mankind's general (but not inborn) condition. It is a distorted and impaired state of disturbed or agitated (vrtti) consciousness (chitta). It is like sun rays passing through coloured glass.
Vrttis attach to the chitta producing vrtti-chitta; that is, resulting in various thought patterns, emotions, feelings, destruction, and agitation. This separates self from its true nature and results in our dualistic nature.

Swami Vivekananda says that **"The chitta, by its own nature, is endowed with all knowledge. It is made of sattva particles, but is covered by rajas and tamas particles; and by pranayama this covering is removed."** (page 181 Raja Yoga)

Yoga can be described as a "tool" of deprogramming this negative conditioning - liberating the individual's modified consciousness from the conditioned consciousness of "non-reality" back into this Original, Natural, and Unmodified state of "Reality".

Thus yoga is a step by step approach by which confused, lonely, destructed, bounded consciousness can be reunited, harmonized, and integrated with its true nature and the Sadhaka can attain intimate sense of belonging in the world, of profound well being, contentment, fulfilment, peace, and joy.
Yoga is aimed to bring us into samadhi (the experience of transpersonal and non-dual union/absorption). Yoga is to attain self- realization called nirbija samadhi (samadhi without seed), wherein even the seeds of future vrttis have become eliminated and dissolved (nirodha) in the state of chitta-vrtti-nirodha.

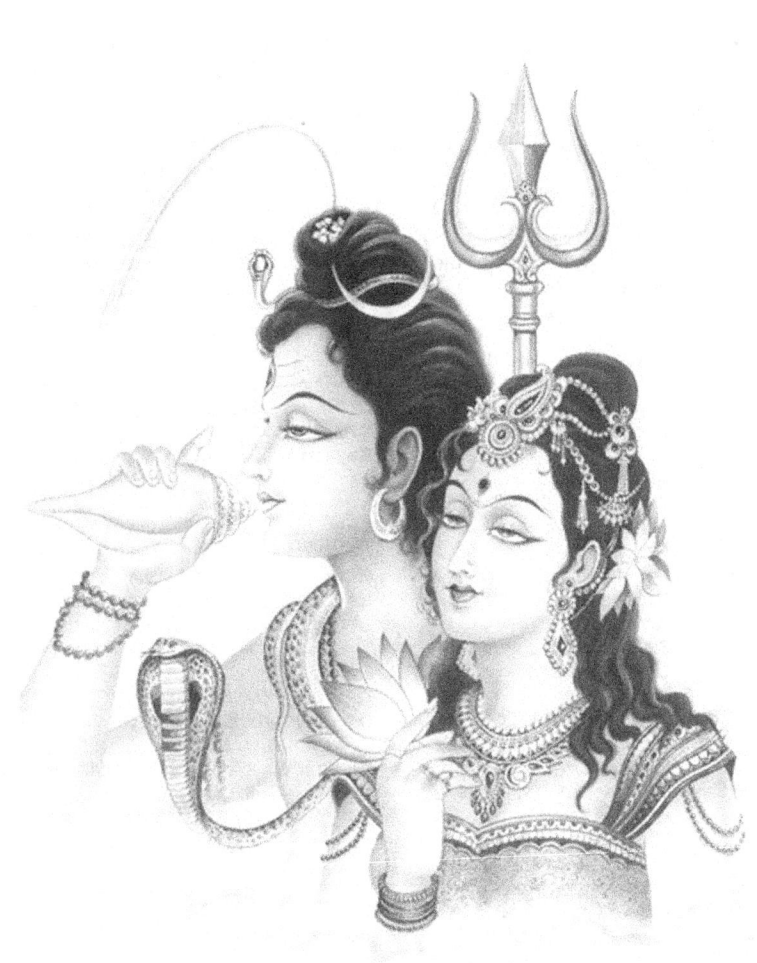

Glossary

Ahamkara ego
Ahimsa Nonviolence, harmlessness (one of the yamas).
Akasha space; ether
Ananda Bliss, joy
Aparigraha Nongreed (one of the yamas).
Arjuna One of the five Pandava back brothers; he whom Lord Krishna Addressed the Bhagavad Gita.
Asanas Yoga postures, 3rd limb of ashtanga yoga.
Ashram Retreat or secluded place, usually where the principles of yoga and meditation are taught and practiced.
Ashtanga Eight limbs
Ashtanga yoga Eightfold path of yoga, Raj Yoga of Patanjali with eight limbs- yamas, Niyamas, etc.
Asmita Ego, individuality, I-am-ness.
Asteya Nonstealing (one of the yamas).
Atma Soul, individual spirit.
Bhakta Devotee.
Bhakti Devotion.
Bhakti yoga The path of devotion.
Brahmacharya Purity, chastity (one of the yamas).
Brahman The absolute. Divinity itself, God as creator.
Buddhi The intellect. Chakras Centers of radiating life force or energy that are located between the base of the spinal column and the crown of the head. Sanskrit for "wheels." There are seven chakras that store and release life force (prana).
Chetana Consciousness, awareness.
Chit Eternal consciousness.
Chit-shakti Mental force governing the subtle dimensions.
Chitta individual consciousness including the subconscious and unconscious levels of mind, memory, thinking, attention, etc.
Chitta-vritti Mental modifications.
Devata Deity
Devi Female deity, goddess.
Dharana From the word dhri meaning "to hold firm," this is concentration or holding the mind to one thought.
Dharma Self-discipline, the life of responsibility and right action.
Dhyana Meditation or contemplation. The process of quieting the mind.
Divya Divine
Doshas Impurities or deformities in body, mind or emotions.
Drashta Seer, observer, awareness.
Drishti Vision.
Gayatri Mantra Vedic mantra of 24 matras or syllables invoking the pure eternal energy.
Gheranda Samhita Traditional yogic text of Rishi Gheranda.
Guru Spiritual teacher.
Hatha yoga It is the yoga of physical well-being, designed to balance body, mind, and spirit.
Indriyas Sense organs.
Ishvar-pranidhana Surrender to God (one of the niyamas).
Iyengar yoga This yoga style focuses on the body and how it works. It is noted for attention to detail, precise alignment of postures, and the use of props.
Jiva Individual life
Jivan Life.
Jnana Knowledge or wisdom.
Jnana yoga The path of knowledge or wisdom.
Kaivalya State of consciousness beyond quality.
Kala Time.
Kama Desires.
Karma Action, law of cause and effect which shapes the destiny of each individual.
Karma yoga The path of action.

Karmendriyas Five physical organs of action- feet, hands, speech, excretory and reproductive organs.
Kirtan Singing holy songs.
Koshas Body, sheaths.
Kriya Motion, movement
Kundalini A cosmic energy in the body that is often compared to a snake lying coiled at the base of the spine, waiting to be awakened. Kundalini is derived from kundala, which means a "ring" or "coil."
Kundalini yoga Chanting and breathing are emphasized over postures in this ancient practice designed to awaken and control the release of kundalini energy.
Laya To dissolve.
Laya yoga Yoga of conscious dissolution of individuality.
Lokas Seven planes of consciousness.
Lord Krishna Because of his great Godly power, Lord Krishna is another of the most commonly worshipped deities in the Hindu faith. He is considered to be the eighth avatar of Lord Vishnu. Shree Krishna delivered Bhagvad Gita on battlefield of Mahabharata to Arjun.
Mala Garland.
Manas Mind.
Mandala A circular geometric design that represents the cosmos and the spirit's journey. It is a tool in the pilgrimage to enlightenment.
Mantra Sacred chant words.
Mauna Silence.
Maya Illusion.
Mitahara Balanced diet.
Moksha Liberation.
Mudras Hand gestures that direct or control the life current through the body.
Mukti Liberation.
Nada Pranic or psychic sound.
Nadi Channels of pranic/psychic energy flow.
Namaste This Hindu salutation says "the divine in me honors the divine in you." The expression is used on meeting or parting and usually is accompanied by the gesture of holding the palms together in front of the bosom.
Nidra Sleep.
Nirbija Samadhi Final state of smadhi where there is absorption without seed; total dissolution.
Nirvichar Samadhi Transitional state of Samadhi; absorption without reflection.
Nirvikalpa Samadhi Transitional state of Samadhi involving purification of memory, which gives rising to Jnana or true knowledge.
Niyamas In the Yoga Sutras, Patanjali defined five niyamas or observances relating to inner discipline and responsibility. They are purity, contentment, self-discipline, study of the sacred text, and living with the awareness of God.
Om or Aum Mantric word chanted in meditation. Paramahansa Yogananda called it the "vibration of the Cosmic Motor." This one word is interpreted as having three sounds representing creation, preservation, and destruction.
Pancha-klesha Five afflictions – ignorance, ego, attraction, aversion and fear of death.
Patanjali Ancient Rishi who codified the ashtanga yoga known as Yoga-Sutra.
Prakriti Nature.
Prana Life energy, life force, or life current vital energy; inherent vital force pervading every dimension of matter.
Pranava Mantra AUM; primal sound vibration.
Pranava Dhyana Meditation on the mantra AUM.
Pranayama Method of controlling prana or life force through the regulation of breathing.

Pratyahara Withdrawing the senses in order to still the mind as in meditation.
Purusha Individual Soul or spirit.
Raja yoga The path of physical and mental control.
Rishi Realised sage, one who meditate on Self.
Sabeeja Samadhi Absorption with seed where the form of awareness remains.
Sadhaka Spiritual aspirant.
Sadhana Spiritual practice.
Sahaja Spontaneous, easy.
Santosha Contentment (one of the niyamas).
Satya Truthfulness and honesty (one of the yamas).
Samadhi State of absolute bliss, superconsciousness (8th limb of ashtanga yoga).
Shaucha Purity, inner and outer cleanliness (one of the niyamas).
Shat-darshanas Six Ancient Indian philosophies about truth or reality.
Swadhyaya Self-study. The process of inquiring into your own nature, the nature of your beliefs, and the nature of the world's spiritual journey (one of the niyamas).
Swami Title of respect for a spiritual master.
Tamas One of the three gunas; state of inertia or ignorance
Tantra yoga This yoga uses visualization, chanting, asana, and strong breathing practices to awaken highly charged kundalini energy in the body.
Tapas Self-discipline or austerity (one of the niyamas). Upanishads. Vedantic texts conveyed by ancient sages and seers containing their experiences and teachings on the ultimate reality.
Vairagya Non-attachment.
Vaisheshika A treatise on the subtle, causal and atomic principles in relation to the five elements.
Vaishnava One who worships Vishnu in the form of Rama, Krishna, Narayana etc.
Vidya Knowledge.
Vijnana Intuitive ability of mind; higher understanding
Vinyasa Steady flow of connected yoga postures linked with breath work in a continuous movement. For example: sun salutation.
Vayu Wind, prana.
Viveka Reasoning and discerning mind; right knowledge or understanding.
Vritti Circular movement of consciousness; mental and modifications described in raja yoga
Yamas In the Yoga Sutras, Patanjali defined five yamas or ways to relate to others — moral conduct. They are nonviolence; truth and honesty; nonstealing; moderation; and nonpossessiveness.
Yantra Visual form of mantra used for concentration and meditation
Yoga Derived from the Sanskrit word for "yoke" or "join together." Essentially, it means union. It is the science of uniting the individual soul with the cosmic spirit.
Yoga nidra Technique of yogic or psychic sleep which induces deep relaxation
Yogi Someone who practices yoga.
Yogini A female yoga practitioner.

www.ingramcontent.com/pod-product-compliance
Lightning Source LLC
Chambersburg PA
CBHW050547300426
44113CB00012B/2293